I0435550

Beauty Revealed

Discover Extraordinary Secrets from Makeup Artists

Table Of Contents

Introduction

Thank you for downloading this book, Beauty Revealed. This book contains tips and tricks to teach you how to do your makeup like the pros. You'll discover how contouring and the elusive smoky eye work and what tools you need to do all of it. Learn the secrets of good skin care and what will make your beauty shine. Don't worry if you've got aging skin, there's information for that too!

Here's an inescapable fact, women are expected to look beautiful. Society judges a woman for how she looks. If you're not a natural beauty then it's almost deemed that you're not worthy or worthless because of it. It sounds misogynistic but it's true. Even women think less of other women who aren't pretty. Studies have shown that the better looking you are the more likely you are to land a job, have a mate, and be successful. No matter how much we protest that it isn't about looks it still makes a difference.

Thankfully, for those that do not wake up model perfect in the mornings there is makeup. In the 1600's makeup was deemed witchcraft because it could transform a woman's beauty. In fact, there have been many Internet challenges that highlight just this effect. Even if you've been doing your makeup for years you may not be doing it justice. If you do not develop your skills constantly your look can become tired, old, and out of date. Like any industry, beauty is constantly evolving. From the sweeping eyeliner popular today to Twiggy's iconic lashes, makeup is always changing. It's time for you to become well versed in how makeup can transform your look.

A good beauty regime covers making your skin as beautiful as possible, without needing makeup. Makeup should be used to enhance this which is what will truly reveal your beauty rather than creating a false image. By knowing your own skin and beauty is what shines through you'll feel better and look more radiant than ever. Beauty isn't just about makeup though it can hide a lot of your flaws. Your face might not be perfect but there are many things you might be doing that can damage your skin. A beautiful makeup look can only cover so much, if your skin is suffering underneath it then you need to fix that as well. Not only will it make applying makeup a lot easier but it will also boost your confidence. Confidence can boost your looks just that little extra and make you truly shine from within.

Chapter 1 – Before You Start

Have you ever looked at your makeup drawer and thought about how much of it you ever wear? Most of us hoard makeup for years, wearing maybe one color out of a palette of ten. Your makeup drawer says a lot about who you are, and it's not just because of the colors you wear. If you're working with a chaotic box with old tissues, used cotton buds, and makeup that you've had since high school then it's time to pull all of it out.

If you've got bottles of concealer and foundation because you've got skin problems but you've had that same bottle for years it might actually be causing the problem! Makeup has an expiration date the same as food. The reason makeup can expire is that it is an ideal place for unhealthy bacteria to grow and build up. When you touch the brushes and applicators to your skin you'll take away a minute amount of dead skin cells. These can get left behind in the palette and will basically just sit and rot. This happens on such a microscopic level you'll never see it. Think of it as an old nail polish bottle that has separated, you can see that the polish has degraded so it's time to throw it away. Your makeup is no different.

Out with the Old

Start by looking at how long you've had everything, throw out grotty looking applicators and pads. Your applicators need to be washed frequently to prevent build up. Disposable sponges should be thrown out after every use, and so should the one that comes with the makeup. These latex pads are ideal places for bacteria to breed and cannot be washed clean enough to be worthwhile. They're also very cheap. A great way of keeping track of your products is to simply write the date on the outside. Here is how long you should keep your makeup before buying new:

- **Mascara – 3 months**. The reason this life is so short is because it starts to dry out quickly. Many people will add saliva or water to thin it back out but all this is doing is introducing bacteria and creating a good chance of having an eye infection.

- **Eye Pencils – 2 years.** If you're sharpening your pencils before each use then you're creating a clean surface which is why these last so long.

- **Eye Shadow – 1-2 years.** Powder shadow will stay fresh longer than a liquid shadow, but if you've had an eye infection or a virus anytime since you bought it and have used your makeup then you need to throw it away. There's a good chance that whatever bacteria caused the infection could still be inhabiting your shadows and may cause it to come back.

- **Lipstick – 2 years.** Just as with eye pencils if you're cleaning off the surface before each use then you're minimizing bacteria.

- **Blush/Powder – 2 years.** Regardless of being cream or powder, these are often the only piece of makeup where you can see and smell the deterioration.

- **Foundation/Concealer – 1 year.** Because we use these directly on fresh skin or with fingers there's a higher chance of these deteriorating fast. If you are using a clean brush each time you can minimize the exposure of your makeup to bacteria and will help lengthen the life of your product.

The Right Tools

Now that you've made some space you can look at your tools. You've probably used the same makeup brushes for years. You bought a kit with 10 brushes and you've only ever used 3. In fact, you probably don't even know what some of them are for. Makeup brushes have very specific uses. That's not to say you're going to need them all, but the fact is having the right brushes to do your makeup can make a huge difference in how well it is applied. Even cheap brushes can do a good job if they're used right. Size really does matter when it comes to brushes, but even though they may be referred to by the type of makeup that you normally use them with they can still have multiple uses. There are some "must have's" when it comes to your brush selection.

Foundation Brush
The foundation brush is a large brush with a flat top. It allows you to place the tip flat to the skin to make the circular motion needed to apply foundation correctly. The brush is especially important if you use powder foundation as it helps to keep that dusting of loose particles to a minimum. They're also more hygienic than sponges or fingers.

Concealer Brush
This is a medium sized brush that has an oval tip. It is usually fairly firm so that you have good control over it. The bristles on a concealer brush are also usually softer (if you're buying good quality brushes and not a one size kit). Since blemishes are usually the result of bacteria it's imperative to clean and wash this after every use.

Powder Brush

The powder brush is similar in size to the foundation brush

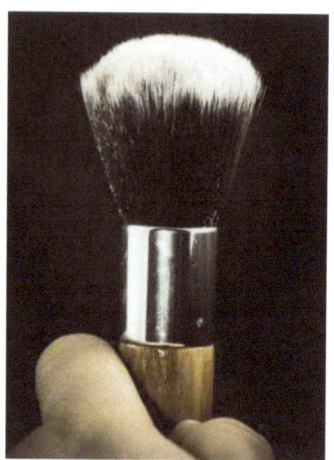

but it has a rounded top. You don't want to confuse the two as putting the top of the powder brush flat to the skin will damage the way the bristles lay. These aren't always a necessity if you're working with powder foundation but they can be very useful for light, overall coverage.

Blush Brush

This is a very important brush, but it's so often overlooked for the powder brush. The blush brush is smaller and usually domed or curved at the tip. The longer bristles give you the ability to have more control over the application area without affecting the foundation or cream underneath. Ideal for applying bronzer, blusher, and also for contouring.

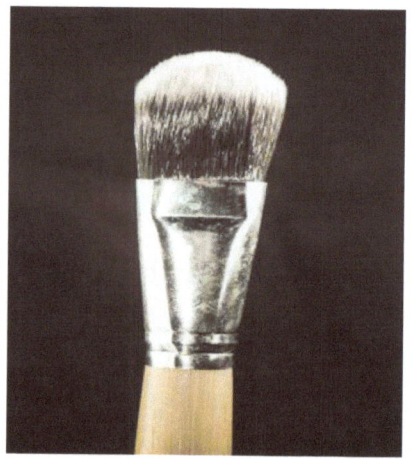

Shadow Brush

Anytime you apply shadow you want to be using one of these.

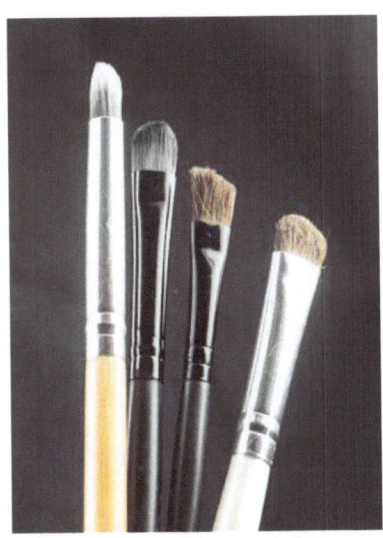

Shadow brushes come in a variety of shapes and sizes so there is no definitive "shadow" brush. What you don't want is to use those nasty foam buds on a stick, you might as well use a cotton swap, throw them away. Since shadow brushes come in many sizes it's a good idea to has a selection of them. Short, long, stiff, soft, etc. Three different ones is a basic minimum for most eyeshadow effects. A soft and stiff brush will help put solid color all over the area. A small and fluffy brush will work best for delicate eyelid and under eye areas. A dome-shaped brush will help to blend everything together.

Angled Liner

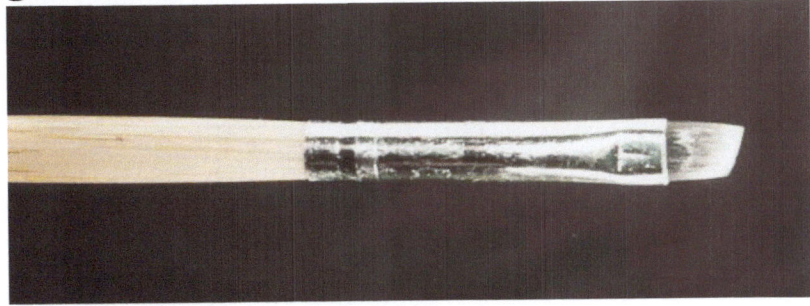

This is more of a mulch-purpose brush as it's too thick for applying eyeliner without looking like a panda. What you need this brush for is brows since it is delicate enough to trace the area without being too big. Look for a firmer brush for brow use. You can still use this brush for a thick liner if you're

7

confident in how steady your hand is. The angle of the brush is deliberate, it's the perfect angle for sweeping across the eyelid in a single motion, with the right liner product this motion can be easy and effective for a thick sweeping line.

Lip Brush

Most of us are guilty of having applied lipstick direct to the skin. This brush is a far better and more sanitary option. The brush works in two ways – the flat and the point. The flat is ideal for large coverage while the point can be used to make precise edges.

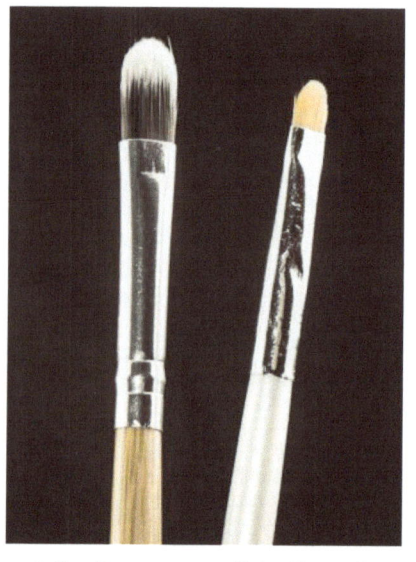

Brow Comb/Spoolie brush

Undoubtedly this is one of the most neglected brushes. Who uses this?? The reason you need this brush is actually very simple. When applying liner, it's common for lashes to clump or stick, because this brush is clean and doesn't have clumps of mascara to add to the problem it can separate lashes out. The brush can also be used to finish the eyebrows and separate the brow hairs.

This is by far the short, short list. Most makeup artists have tens of brushes in their toolkit. If you're not looking to go pro then these are the basic minimum. You'll also need a few sponge applicators if you want a more solid look to your foundation. It's also a good idea to have other tools like an eyelash curler in your arsenal. Most makeup artists use false eyelashes but it's important to curl your own to match if you want a flawless look.

Cleaning

Chances are by now you're looking at your brushes and thinking how disgusting they are. If you're not buying new ones then you'll need to clean them. Cleaning brushes after each use is an important part of applying great makeup. No professional uses dirty brushes, it's unsanitary and it won't provide the best result. If you want to buy some liquid brush cleaner and you can start by massaging some into the bristles before rinsing them off. Most professionals use brush cleaner every time they're finished with their brushes and will shampoo them between clients for sanitation purposes.

To clean your brushes, you'll need a clean towel, very hot water, baby shampoo (Dawn will also work), and a sink. First run the brushes under warm water with the bristles pointing downwards. You want the gunk to run off the brush not back up into the handle. Massage the bristles gently to separate them and make sure the water saturates the head. Place a small amount of shampoo into your hand and swirl the bristles around into the shampoo (as if you were using the brush to collect makeup). Once the brush is lathered up pinch the bristles at the head and squeeze the liquid out in a downward motion. Rinse and repeat until the water runs clear. With a clean paper towel pat the brush dry and make sure the end if formed back to it's original shape. Lay the brush out on a clean towel to dry and make sure they are thoroughly dry overnight before using. Drying is just as important as washing since a wet brush may mold if left damp.

Chapter 2 – Preparing the Skin

You only have one face, it has to be with you for the rest of your life so you should take care of it. It takes about size months before you see significant improvement in your skin but you may see some results within a week if your routine hasn't been working. Any good makeup artist will tell you that taking care of your skin first makes makeup a whole lot easier. Not only that but with good skin you're going to need less of it. Cleaning your brushes and throwing out old products is a good start in your skincare routine. Just as your brushes need to be washed so too does your skin. During the day (and night) your skin secretes oils and sheds dead skin cells. The last thing you want to be doing before putting makeup on is pushing all this back into your pores. Before even thinking of putting makeup on you need to wash your skin.

Cleaning and Scrubbing

Exfoliation is important if you want to scrub the muck off. Much of the reason your skin doesn't seem to "glow" is because this takes fresh skin cells. Don't forget your neck and decolletage area, many people concentrate on the face and this area is neglected, it will show. The dead skin on the surface is often what causes makeup to be flaky and look dry. By exfoliating regularly, you're helping to encourage dead skin cells to start the shedding process and the fresh cells to reproduce and form more skin cells. This will also encourage the skin cells production of both collagen and elastin, both of these nutrients help skin to appear younger. You should exfoliate at least once a week, but not every day as this can cause your skin to toughen and dry out.

It's a horrible idea to sleep in your makeup, you're simply asking for break outs. Before heading to bed always remove your makeup. Look for a cleanser that is pH-balanced, your skin is naturally slightly acidic to fight off bacteria so you want to retain that. Make sure you're rinsing off properly afterward so no residue remains. If your skin is sensitive you need to avoid products that contain hydroxyl or glycolic acids as these can dry the skin and cause irritation.

Moisturizer

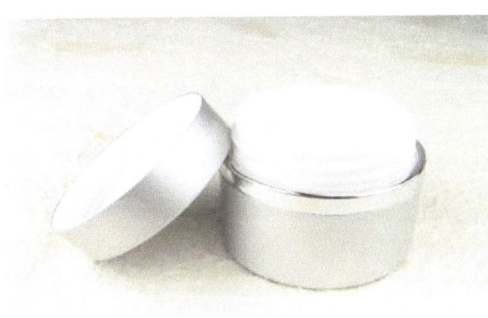

Your skin can dry out overnight so it's important that it is clean and hydrated before bed. Make sure you're applying a moisturizer before bed that has retinol in. Retinol helps to stimulate skin cells and collagen for plumper looking skin. You'll also need moisturizer for daytime use too. This can be as important since the wrong moisturizer will form an oily barrier on your skin and your makeup will literally slide off. It's a prudent idea to also apply an overnight skin serum with your moisturizer as this will help rejuvenate the cells with important vitamins and minerals to keep the upper layers of skin cells healthy.

Most dermatologists agree that using moisturizer is the number one most important part of any skincare routine after cleansing. Without moisturizer your skin forms micro-cracks between skin cells as it dries, this is an ideal place for bacteria to get in and for your skin to start to age. It's not even a secret, we all know we should moisturize properly but few of us do it regularly.

The best moisturizer to wear under makeup is one that doesn't make your makeup look caked on or so oily that it slides off. Try and stay away from ones that are intended for acne use unless you really need them. The reason you want to do this is that with regular use the chemicals used to treat acne will just dry the skin cells out, doing the opposite of what you need. Excessive drying can actually make the problem worse. Look for one that is oil-free to avoid the sliding effect. Applying your moisturizer and allow it to soak in properly before starting on your makeup will really make a difference in how well your skin looks and how well the makeup goes over it.

Sunscreen

Sunscreen is also extremely important. The sun will age and damage your skin like nothing else, and your face is constantly being exposed. Many modern makeup products have an included sun protection factor but if yours doesn't it's important to know how to put that on under your makeup. In fact, many advertised products that have sunscreen in them expect you to use 10 times the normal amount to reach that protection factor so it's a good idea to simply add sunscreen to your pre-makeup routine anyway. Many sunscreens are oily in nature so you want to find one that has a natural feel and soaks into your skin properly. An oily barrier will make it difficult to apply your makeup well. You can also look for moisturizers that have built in sunscreen so that you're not using too much. If you're using both moisturize first.

Once your face is clean apply the sunscreen liberally over your face and neck (seriously, no one remembers the neck area!).

You'll also want to apply SPF balm over your lips and allow it to soak in. Make sure you've covered your whole face including the hairline and as close to your eyes as you can. Consider adding a spray on transparent misting sunscreen to your day bag as this will allow you to reapply, and reset your makeup without having to touch it up.

Now that your skin is prepared you can look at applying your base layers. Without a clean and well-prepared canvas makeup often doesn't last as long or can be difficult to apply. If you've ever struggled to get rid of that cake-like look or had your eyeshadow dissolve into the creases then you're not applying your base or doing the right prep.

Shaving

It's a hot debate whether you should or shouldn't shave your face. The tiny little hairs on your face do affect how well your makeup lays on there, and they are what can make it look too heavy. Some women feel that the more you shave the more hair will grow back, rather like a man's face. It's actually a bit of a fallacy. You only need to razor your face if you really feel you need it. If you're thinking of shaving, buying a razor which is specifically designed for use on facial hair is also a prudent idea. Facial razors look nothing like your man's razor and nothing like your leg razors. They are different to avoid this whole problem and to give you more precise control. If you feel you need to shave then do so before washing your skin, you'll want the skin to have time to recover before applying makeup so that it isn't irritated.

Healthy Skin

Healthy skin starts from within. If your diet is poor then it might be causing the majority of the problems you're trying to hide with makeup. Good hydration is essential for beautiful skin so try and keep hydrated with a minimum of 8 glasses of water a day. It might seem a lot but your body uses water for most of its processes and without enough of it our cells start to suffer. One of the first places you'll notice dehydration is your skin. Depending on what your dietary issues are there are often signs on your skin. Your face ,for example, will break out in certain areas relating to your hormones, too much fat in the diet, or because your liver is overburdened with toxins. Take some time to adjust your diet and see how your skin improves. Exercise can also help by improving the blood flow in the body.

Chapter 3 – Makeup 101: Color Theory

When it comes to makeup most of us want to go color crazy. The key to having successful color combinations is to know your natural skin tones and accentuate them. You'll also need to know how to get rid of any unwanted color. You might open your primer up and find out that it's green. Having a green primer removes redness in the skin tone since the red cancels out the green. Colors can be divided up into ones that cancel each other out or that accentuate each other. This is a color wheel:

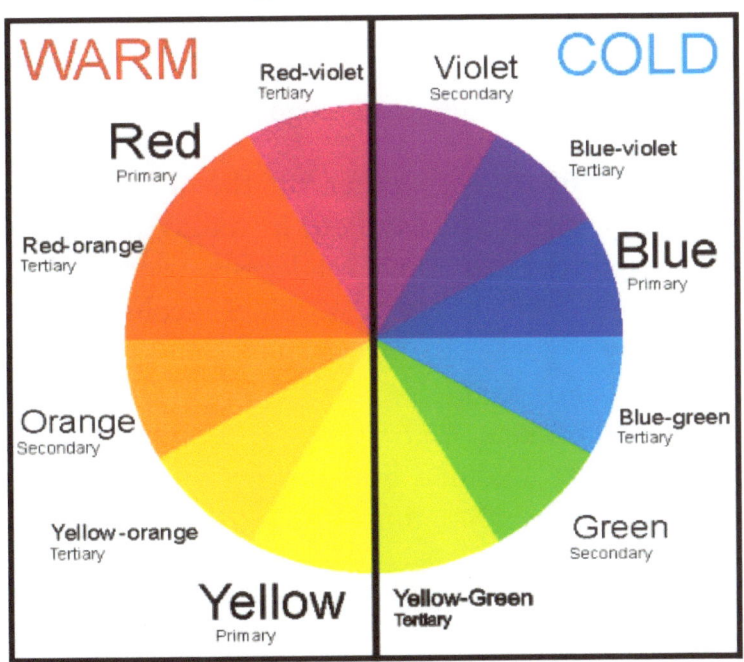

As you can see red and green are opposite each other. Colors that are opposites cancel each other out or accentuate each other if they are adjacent. Color theory is makeup 101. Each color has it's own feel and it's own result. Certain colors will make a statement, evoke a mood, or even make another color go away. Basic color theory is knowing what will happen when you place different colors on top of each other or next to each other and what the influence will be. Some of the most common questions that makeup artists hear are "What colors look good on me?" and "Why don't I look good in this shade?".

Color Theory

Colors are broken down into Primary, Secondary, and Tertiary colors. There are three primary colors: yellow, red and blue. They are called primary colors because they cannot be mixed by making other colors. Secondary colors are made by mixing any two of these primary tones like green or orange. Tertiary colors are mixed by combining any secondary color and a primary color. Colors can then be broken down into complementary or analogous. Analogous colors are those

that are adjacent to each other on the color wheel while complimentary colors are any two, including primary colors, which are opposite each other. Analogous colors will create a similar scheme and enhance a single color tone while complimentary colors will make each tone stand out with better contrast. For example, having a green eyeshadow with red lipstick will make both colors into a bold statement. Similarly, wearing a golden toned eyeshadow with blue eyes will create the same contrasting effect.

When complimentary colors are mixed they will create a neutral beige tone. Many processes such as foundation and concealer work through the process of color theory. A great example of this is green concealer. The green tone cancels out the red from a blemish leaving it a neutral tone that can easily blend in with the makeup around it. We'll look at neutral tones further on.

All the colors can also be broken down into warm and cool tones. When it comes to your skin you'll frequently see people saying they have warm or cool toned skin or referring to a season that has similar colors in the palette, "I've got winter tones" etc. It's important to match the makeup to these tones or you'll end up with a contrasting look that isn't altogether appealing. A common misconception is that all blonde people have cool tone skin and all dark skin tones are warm. There's a good chance that if you're struggling to match your skin color properly you're looking in the wrong color section.

Skin Tones

Skin tones are divided into warm, neutral and cool. Cool skin tones have a slight pink tone and tend to be people who burn easily in sunlight. These are also people who look good in silver jewelry and maybe have visible blue veins under the skin. Warm skin tones are those who have a golden tone to the skin, they usually look better with gold accessories and tend to have almost a greenish tint to their veins. Warm tones tend to look washed out in cool colors. Those with a neutral tone of skin tend to be able to pull off any look, they can wear gold or silver and have a mixture of both rosy and golden looks in their skin.

When it comes to buying makeup start by trying to figure out if your skin is warm or cool and match your colors accordingly. This can be especially important when it comes to concealer. Concealer application can be one of the most difficult parts of flawless makeup, too orange and it sticks out, too pale and it looks obvious. Recently there have been several tutorials showing girls putting lipstick under their eyes to better hide dark circles. The reason this works is because the cold blue tone of the skin is canceled out by the orange of the lipstick. Color theory applies even before you start picking out colors.

Color Correcting

The process of fixing and canceling out colors is known as color correcting. It's one of the most underused things in everyday makeup. Most people don't even know about it. There are 5 things you can use a color correcting palette for. You probably don't need all of them but you'll more than likely suffer from one or two of these. The color correcting palette is something you should use alongside contouring and good base application. It's similar to contouring as it's creating an image of what should be there by hiding what you don't want to see. Here are the 5 different ways you can use complimentary colors to correct issues in your skin tone:

Redness: Ideal for zits, overly rosy cheeks or hiding pink scars you'll want a green tone to cancel out the red. You can use green primer or concealer for this purpose.

Yellow/sallow skin: Many ethnic tones have a yellow undertone that can look almost unhealthy. Using a primer that has a purple tone to it can brighten the skin up and bring it to a nice neutral shade.

Dull Skin: If your skin looks somewhat tired then it probably has a blueish tint to it. Using a yellow tinted powder will brighten it right up.

Brown Circles under the eye: Some people have blueish bags while others have brown. Depending on your skin tone if you have brown looking bags under the eyes you'll want to add a cool pink tone. This is one of the reasons that the web hack of red lipstick works for many people, once blended it creates the perfect pink tone. Using a pink will also help brighten the eye area once that brown is canceled out.

Blue Circles under the Eye: If you're one of the people with blue under eye tones then choose a peachier or orange corrector. If you add a pink undertone you'll often find they don't go away fully. Blue undertones need a warm complimentary color (orange) to become neutral, pink is the wrong color as it isn't warm enough.

Neutral Tones

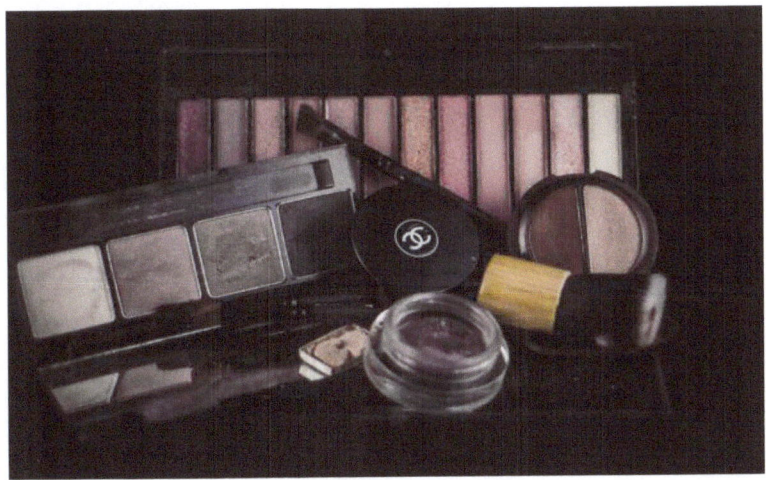

Neutral tones are neither warm nor cool, most foundations are neutral toned so that they can blend with as many skin tones as possible. The biggest benefit of neutrals is they are ideal for background or understated looks that work for everyone. If you look at a neutral toned palette you'll probably think it looks warm, since neutral colors are affected by the colors around them they usually reflect whatever stronger color they are paired with. Black, white, and cream are the strongest neutral tones. It's a very good idea to have at least one palette of nude or neutral color tones to work with to create everyday looks.

Monochrome

Monochrome schemes use analogous colors. All the colors come from the same color "family" - reds, blues, yellows, greens etc. These are the simplest color arrangements and are ideal for matching and creating a simple but effective color scheme. They're also great if you're not very confident with color theory as you'll be able to match products easier. The outstanding thing about a monochrome palette is that you can combine textures to get arresting effects. For example, shiny, matte, shimmer, cream, and velvet. When using a monochrome of neutral tones, the look is referred to as nude. Nude is a classy yet impressive look that suits any skin tone but it can be difficult to pull off if your palette isn't quite close enough.

Color Meanings

On top of all this, colors can have their own feel. Most colors have a "feel" to them, this means they will evoke a feeling or memory just by using them. For example, a woman in red lipstick is usually deemed "sexy" because red is a color that evokes lust. When choosing a color palette to wear you'll often evoke a certain response from those around you just by picking one color over another. This is true whether you're talking about clothes, makeup or even the walls of your house. Some colors and combinations will also evoke certain holidays – for example, red and green for Christmas. Here is the list of color meanings:

- Red – Love, Lust, Passion, Sexy, Anger, Violence

- Orange – Energy, Vitality, Autumn

- Yellow – Hope, Sunshine, Happiness, Youth, Summer

- Green – Nature, Growth, Zen, Balance, New Beginnings

- Blue – Calm, Focus, Depth, Sadness, Winter

- Purple – Royalty, Wealth, Power, Wisdom, Creativity

- Pink – Youth, Sweetness, Naivete, Purity

- White – Clean, Virtue, Purity, Light, Winter

- Grey – Blank, Conservative, Dull,

- Black – Mystery, Evil, Elegance, Power, Death,

- Brown – Nature, Autumn, Dependable,

Now you're ready to start applying your makeup. Hopefully you're enjoying this book, if so share your thoughts and post a review. It'd be greatly appreciated!

Chapter 4 – Foundation & Contouring

Now that your skin is prepared and you've figured out your color palette you're ready to apply base. Your skincare routine should not leave your face feeling oily, if your skin feels oily then blot it with oil cloths or a paper towel before continuing. Many people find applying the base layer of makeup the most confusing. Should you conceal first or contour first? Do you need foundation if you're contouring? Do you even need primer? All very good questions. In fact, most products will go back and forth in a layering process depending on what sort of look you're going for. It can even be a hassle picking out the right tone. One of the craziest thing you'll hear is that if you're picking color shades is to stop using the back of your hand! Use the inside of your arm as it more closely resembles your facial skin.

Primer

If you're an average girl there's a huge chance you've never bought primer. Primer is one of the biggest and foremost secrets in makeup but very few ordinary women use it which means they are truly missing out. Primer can be an absolute godsend if you're not keen on adding a full face of makeup. Most people skip this step feeling it's unnecessary or because they don't want to invest in a product they're not familiar with. What primer does it that it acts as a base for foundation and it acts as a preparation for makeup to stick to. It really helps the makeup to adhere, giving you a smoother and more flawless look. You can buy specific primers like eyelid primer, or one that has mattifying properties if you're prone to oilier skin. If you really want your makeup to stay put then primer is a must.

Primer can be applied using a sponge or fingertips, it needs to be applied in a circular motion and really worked into the skin. Consider applying primer as an exercise in massage that also stimulates the skin cells and improves blood flow to them. If you're not keen on applying too many layers just applying primer alone can make your skin seem a lot fresher and polished compared to bare skin. It's very much the "natural look" without actually going natural. Not all primers are skin tone. Don't worry if your primer is green, it's meant to either provide sheer coverage or just as a preparation for color. The green tone will remove redness in your skin tone. You'll also be applying it over your powder (trust us).

If you don't have primer but are prone to oily skin, in a pinch you can add a dusting of corn starch before applying foundation.

Blemishes

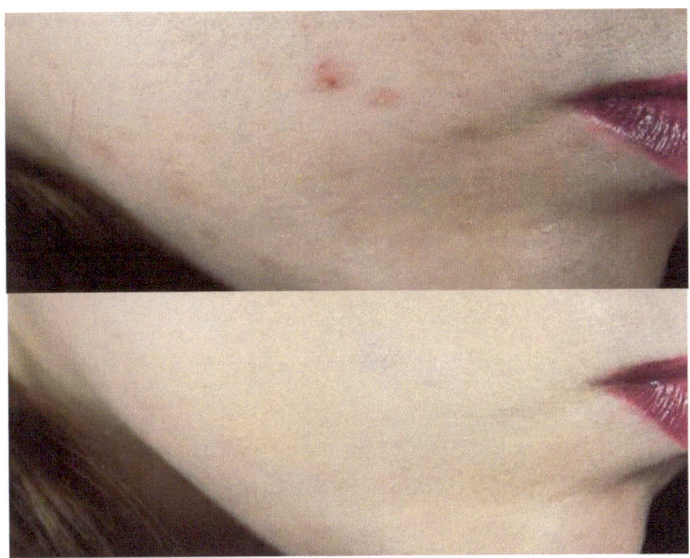

Concealer goes on first, and third. Confusing right? The reason you want to apply layers of concealer is so that it blends in well with everything else. Chances are you've got one that is close to your skin tone, but even if it's close it might still be a shade off from your foundation and blending it will thin the coverage so that it shows through. Apply concealer after foundation to stop creasing in the area. Try and blend the edges seamlessly by applying to a slightly larger area and only blending the edges. Powder over the blemishes to set this layer before continuing. You can also choose to powder the entire face at this time as it will add an extra layer of coverage.

Before applying foundation, you can also apply blush if you choose. Blush tends to scare people, they don't want to look like a clown, but they don't want to be without it either. A great way around the problem is to put it on before foundation. If you're not confident enough to put it on after putting blush on before foundation will give you an inner glow rather than an icing look.

Foundation

Foundation is the base of all your makeup, it needs to be strong so that everything else will stay in place. How you apply foundation is a bit of a debate among professionals. Some will swear by their brushes while others insist on using sponges. The reason that I'm not a fan of sponges is that they soak up the oils and foundation itself meaning you're not getting the full product on your skin, just what the sponge leaves on the top. Try both and decide for yourself if necessary but I'm firmly on the side of good brushes. If you're planning on contouring you'll need a good cream foundation, it's much easier to blend and will give enough coverage, unlike powder.

To apply the foundation use small amounts at a time, around a dime size. Squeeze the foundation onto the back of your hand and then dip the brush tip in. Using circular motions press the foundation into your skin with a firm stroke. This applies for both powder and liquid. Use the flat face of the brush not the edge. One of the biggest tricks to the perfect foundation is applying only the coverage you need. Once upon a time, we had to cake foundation all over. The only time this works with modern makeup is by blending it all over, including the eye is to create an airbrushed effect. If you're piling it on because you know you'll be photographed it's quite unnecessary since modern cameras are less likely to wash your skin out. For an everyday look, all you will need is a few dabs on your T-zone and on areas where you want to camouflage redness.

Concealer

Concealer isn't just for blemishes or the baggies under your eyes. Concealer can really aid in evening out your skins natural variations in tone. If you've got dark spots or areas that have a shadowing to them then liberally applying concealer is an easy way to balance things out. Concealer is an important tool if you're planning on contouring because you need the base layer to be as even as possible all over.

Contouring

The most important part of contouring is knowing how

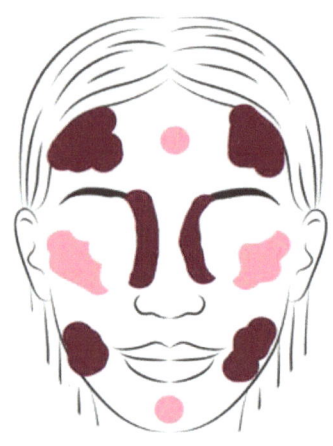

dramatic you need to go. Contour too much and you'll look like a drag queen, contour too little and it won't look like you've done anything. Take a look at this graphic, what you're seeing is a road map to basic contouring.

Contouring is a mixture of dark and highlighting on the face that changes the shape by fooling the eye. Darker areas will recede while highlighted areas will stand forwards. They are equally important. The darker area will give you the contour you need to adjust your face shape while the highlight will make the skin seem fuller and more youthful. Each color on this diagram represents a different makeup on your contour palette. The simplest contour colors are just a bright white and a dark brown, even if you don't have contouring makeup you can make do if you have those. What you want to be aiming for is a shade that is two shades darker and two shades lighter than your natural tone, this will give a more authentic look. Each face shape has different contouring needs. If you're not sure what shape your face is, have a look at this diagram and see. You'll also notice where the suggested highlight and shadow areas are.

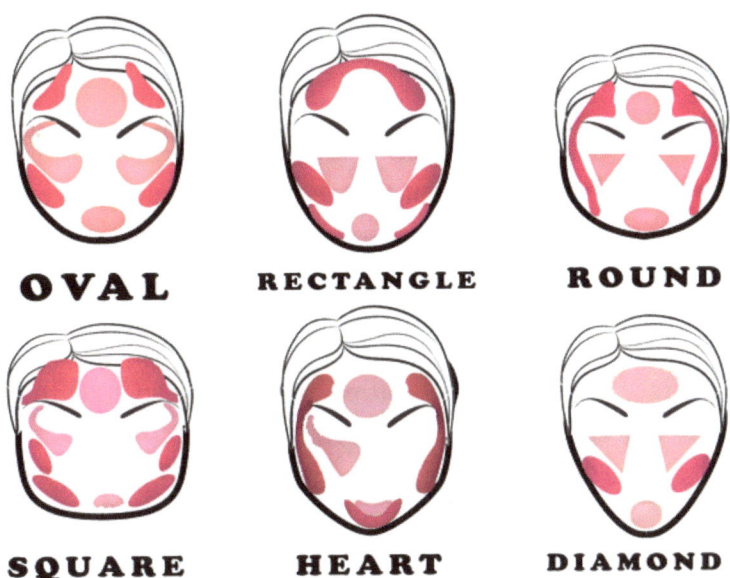

OVAL   **RECTANGLE**   **ROUND**

SQUARE   **HEART**   **DIAMOND**

Diamond Face: The shadowed area below your cheekbones should extend back to the ears but stop in the middle of your cheek (approximately under the pupil of each eye). The highlighted areas should be under the eyes and along the brow bone. Also, apply bright highlights to the ball of the chin and the center of the forehead to create a broader look.

Heart Face: Shadow long the sides of the forehead and temple area to narrow the forehead so that it matches the chin. Contour the cheeks from the ears to the middle of the cheekbone and below the chin so that the chin doesn't appear so sharp. Highlight the area under the eyes and in the middle of the forehead and chin. Make sure to bring the highlighted eye area around to the sides too.

Oblong Face: An oblong face needs to be shortened so contour along the hairline and to the sides of the forehead.

You'll also want to contour the cheekbones and along the jaw where the chin is. Highlight only the area under your eyes and brow to brighten the area.

Oval Face: One of the easiest to contour the oval actually allows you to be more flexible with how severe you want your contouring. Shadow the sides of the forehead and under the cheekbones to add depth. Highlight the chin and forehead as well as around the eye and brow to brighten.

Rectangle Face: Contour along the forehead and hairline to narrow the area, do this right down the sides of the temple and not just at the top but do not go down to the cheekbones. Use the same shade and contour the sides of the jawline to narrow the area. Contour under the cheekbones with a darker shade. Highlight only the chin and under the eyes, you don't want to add width to the forehead.

Round Face: Contour along the temples and all the way down to the jaw line to narrow the face. Bring the contour line in at the cheekbones and at the forehead for a narrower look. Highlight the center of the forehead and chin only. Use a small highlight under the eyes to brighter but do not bring it down too far.

Square Face: One of the most complex to contour, You'll want large shadowed areas at the temples and at the outermost jaw. Bring the contour down under the jawline to make it narrow. You'll also want to add a little contour shadow under the cheekbones but not as heavy and leaving a gap before the jawline. Highlight the middle forehead and chin but focus on the eye area. Use a slightly darker highlight on the forehead. On the eye area make sure you get the top of the cheeks and around to the brows.

Notice not one of these required you to contour your nose? Many people do not need their nose "slimmed" down. Unless you're going for an ultra narrow look like Kim K then you really don't need to worry about contouring your nose. If you think you need it then apply shadow along the sides of your nose with a little across the bridge and half an inch from the tip. Apply highlight between the side lines and a little on the tip. The nose is one of the most difficult parts of the face to contour and to make it appear natural so don't fret if it takes some practice. Now that your face is somewhat evened out you'll also want to reapply concealer to any blemishes that are coming through, blend the concealer the same as before.

Powder

If you want your cheekbones to be very dramatic then save the cheekbone contouring until after you've applied powder. If you want to retain a somewhat blended look then apply powder over the top of your cheekbones. This is also an ideal way of fixing contouring that is too dark – simply apply a lighter powder over the top and blend. You'll want a powder that is a little lighter than your skin tone but not a lot. The trick to applying powder is that after you've applied brush over the whole thing gently so that there is no loose dusting left. Choose an illuminating translucent powder so that your face glows. It's also a good idea to apply it to your eyelids and eye area a little thicker if your dark areas are showing through. Do not go overboard as too light on the eyes is as bad as too dark.

Blush & Bronze

Here's one amazing little trick that really works. After you've powdered but before applying blush take a little of your primer and tap a couple of dabs on top of your cheekbones where you're applying bronzer and blush. What this will make your blush more vibrant and help it last longer. Now the debate comes as to whether you need blusher and bronzer or just one or the other.

Bronzer is intended for creating a tanned look or gentle contour while blusher is for adding a healthy glow. If you're not using your bronzer for contouring then it probably isn't needed. You can use both together. There are two types of bronzer – shimmery and matte. A shimmery bronzer can be dusted over the entire face to create a healthy tanned glow while the matte bronzer is better used for contouring purposes. The key to picking the right bronzer is color. Stick with the two shades darker rule and you won't end up looking like you have dirt on your face. The easiest way to apply bronzer is in the shape of a 3 and reversed. Start the 3 at your temple, dust along the cheek and sweep down to the jawline and across to the chin.

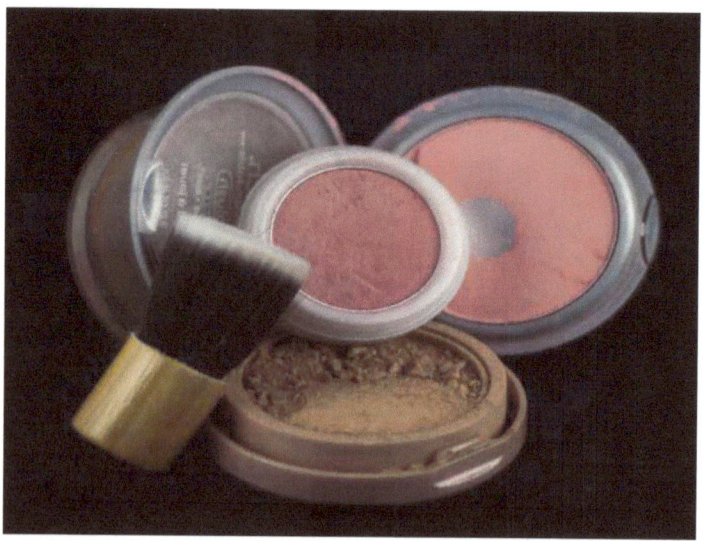

When it comes to applying blush there are two things to keep in mind – your face shape and your blush color. There isn't a right or wrong way to apply blush, it's very dependent on what you want to do. Powder blush has the longest staying powder while tint blushers are only intended for a light flushed look and not really suitable for full makeup. There are four main colors of blush – pink, plum, beige, and peach. You'll actually want to have two shades of blush to get your colors right – one to apply on top that is lighter and one to apply under the cheekbones that is darker. The oranger blush tone should only be applied to the fullest point of the cheek.

PINK: Pink blush should only sit on the apple of your cheek, it's meant to give a rosy look, not an actual shape. The key with pink blush is not to put a lot of it. To find the apple of your cheek grin at the mirror, the apple is the puffy part in the middle between the tip of your lip and the pupil of your eye. Using a medium sized, dome shape brush apply in circles just to the apple area. Do not go into the smile lines or up on the cheekbones.

PLUM: These are often better on darker complexions and can be applied the same as pink blushes, the more rouge like colors should only be used on dark skin or very tan skin.

BEIGE: This is merely to enhance your natural tone, it's meant to add fullness without adding color. You'll want to put beige blush only on the top part of the cheek apple. Using a larger and fuller powder brush apply a veil all over the area. Start at the edge of the cheekbones and work inwards. You'll want to leave the inner third of the cheek apple bare.

PEACH: Peach is a good tone to use with contouring. The reason for this is that it's most often the closest to your natural tones. To find your cheekbone pull your mouth to the side and smirk creating tension along the cheek line. Using an angled brush sweep along the cheekbones dragging the color forward from the ears. If you're not sure you've got the right line then line the brush up with the little flap of skin at the front of your ear and stop at the beginning of your cheek apple. The majority of the color should be back away from the cheek and more on the cheekbones.

When it comes to applying blush for your face shape you'll need to keep your contouring in mind. If you've worked hard on creating sharp cheekbones then stick with sweeping along them to accent them. If you're working with your natural shape use one of these as a template:

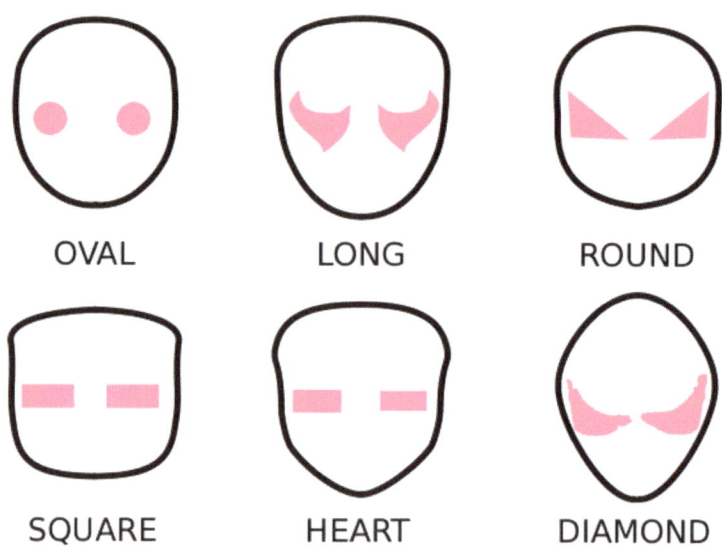

OVAL   LONG   ROUND

SQUARE   HEART   DIAMOND

Chapter 5 – The Eyes

The eyes tend to be the first thing we notice about a person. Your eyes can say a lot of things, they can age you or they can stop a person in their tracks. Eyes are often the most crucial part of your makeup regimen, in fact, many women merely wear mascara and no other products because they know that this is the first and only place another person is guaranteed to look. When it comes to making a statement from your eyes you'll need to consider their color, shape, and what effect you're going for.

Eye Contouring

Eyes can come in many shapes, but what you don't want to do is to make them disappear in a sea of makeup. Your eyes may not even be the same shape as each other. Using makeup to adjust this is important, you can make your eyes stand out simply by making them a better shape for your face. Eye contouring is done similarly to your face but on a much smaller scale. We've already mentioned using color correction to fix dark under eyes, but you'll also need to use With the right adjustments you can fix any flaws in your eye area. Here are a few ways you can contour your eye to change the shape.

- **Definition:** To add more definition to your eye use a bronzer that is only slightly darker than your skin tone. This will help add more definition to the crease, especially if your skin is aging. An orange tone bronzer will also help bring out the blue in your eye color. You can also add definition by applying a black pencil to the upper, inner eyelid rim. What this does is add fullness to the lash line without a sweeping eyeliner outside.

- *A* **Add width:** If your eyes are narrow set you can bring them out by adding a sweep of eye liner to the outer edge of the lashes and connecting them at the edge. This will add a darker area at the end of the eye which will be hard to notice with mascara on (unless you overdo it and make a dramatic wing).

- *A* **Drooping Lids:** as we age our skin loses some its youthful elasticity, causing the skin around the eyelid to drop down. Using the same theory as facial contouring you can fix this. Apply a strong highlight above the crease and then blend a shadow into this from the creased area. By using an eye luminizer at the inner tear duct corner of the eye and drawing it down around the bottom of the eye it will also help brighten the whole face up.

- *A* **Small Eyes:** Using a lighter eyeliner (beige) edge the lower rim so that it is brighter than the skin around, this will make the eye seem wider. Pencil around this on the lower lash line and then along the upper line. Smudge the line outwards to draw the eye along the lash line.

Eye Color

When it comes to color theory we've already seen how important color can be. Your eye color is already there, which means unless you're wearing contacts you're going to have to work with it. Your eye and skin tone will determine the best color palette for your makeup. It's a good idea to think in opposites. By placing the opposite color for your iris color next to it, it will make it stand out more. Remember the gold eyeshadow and blue eyes? This creates a striking effect by using opposites. Similarly, you can also use the same color as your eye tone to create a monochrome effect. When it comes to the three main eye colors (blue, green, brown) you can easily create an impressive look using one color as long as it's the right one.

Blue Eyes: For blue eyes you'll need to pay close attention to your skin tone. If you're working with cool skin tones warm colors may make you seem washed out, and cold colors may make you seem too cold. Make sure your eye color matches with your base makeup or that your base is neutral. The complimentary color of blue is orange, but it's unlikely that you're going to want to have a bright orange shadow. Pick a color that has orange undertones like a gold, apricot or peach. Alternatively, go with shades of blue, white, and teal if you're sticking with a cold palette. This will also work for gray eyes.

Green Eyes: You're just as unlikely to pile on red eyeshadow

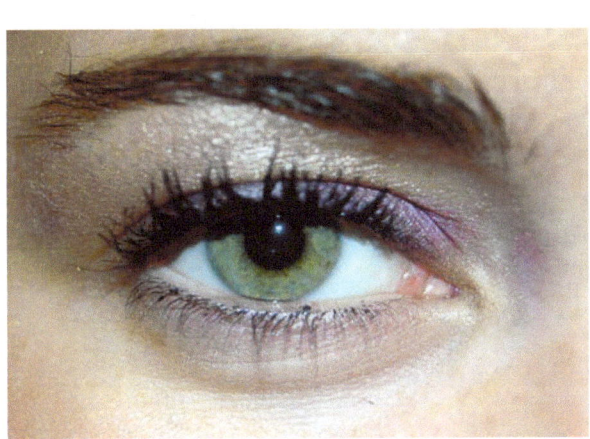 as orange when it comes to green eyes. The look could potentially be striking, or it could be downright scary. Stick to colors that have red undertones in them to bring out the green. You'll also be in a perfect position to use neutral pink tones such as a dusky rose. Colors that have red undertones like plum, deep purple, some pinks, and even a warm brown will work well with green eyes. You can also choose greens or green toned colors like lime, teal, or even gold. Stay away from cold colors as they are unlikely to suit you.

Brown Eyes: Brown is a perfectly neutral color which means you'll be able to get away with just about any color. You can pick one color from both palettes such as a blue and a purple and get very good effects. If you have a brown hazel and want to bring out your secondary color pick the appropriate one from the above.

Eye Brows

Most of us do something to shape our brows. Waxing, plucking, string, there's a good chance your brows are already manicured into a good shape. So why do anything to them? When you're putting on makeup there's a good chance your brows are also getting dusted. Your eyebrow hairs are also unlikely to be as full or defined as you would like. A good brow adds a frame to the eye that helps with facial definition. We've all seen the eyebrow horror story memes, just by making a mess of that one feature the entire face becomes a joke. There are many reasons your eyebrows might be looking a little off when you're applying makeup. It's a prudent idea to be sure that your makeup primer is also blended right into your brow line as this will help the color stay put longer.

Avoid squaring the line of the brow off at the bridge of the nose. We're all guilty of trying to make our brows precision sharp, but this makes them look fake. Using an angled brush or pencil make small strokes that mimic the other hairs and create a softer edge.

If you think back on those eyebrow memes they all have one thing in common, they are exaggerated. Unless you want to find yourself on the same page try not to create an arch that is too high. Your arch should line up with the outside of your nostril. You'll also want to use your spoolie or brow brush to brush the hair downwards to apply your product and then brush them back over when you're done so that it looks more natural.

Usually it's by accident, but many of us suffer from too long eyebrows. You know the story, you try and even them up, then one gets even longer and before you know it your eyebrow goes down a level to the edge of your eye. Having too long of a tail on your eyebrow brings the face down, and it will make you appear sad. To measure where your eyebrow line should stop you need to take a long pencil and line the length of it up from your nose to the outer side of your eye. Where the line of the pencil crosses over with your brow line is the perfect length.

Probably one of the most common mistakes when it comes to eyebrows is using the wrong color. Making your brows too dark will make them seem false, and they will also make you look angry. You want your eyebrows to match your hair unless you're one of those graced with brows that are a completely different color and they you'll need to go with what works with your skin tone. As you age your brows thin and lose color, this is especially important once your hair goes gray as most colors will be too dark to create a positive frame. Black hair is the most difficult to match, you don't want to have black brows, it is too extreme and will wash your skin out. Instead, opt for a dark gray or extremely dark brown. Make sure you're matching your skin tone with a warm or cool color for your eyebrow choice.

Prepping the eye

It seems there are tons of different products you can use for your eyes but what's really the difference? Pencil is a smudgy look that comes in many colors, but it will also need to be sharpened regularly. Don't use a pencil for creating a sharp line but rather for adding a smudged area. A liquid liner tends to last longer and has a more precise and dramatic look. Gel liners are the most daunting for most people, they require special brushes and may dry much quicker than any other type. They're a good combination of both though since you can smudge or create sharp lines.

You can buy specific eyelid primer but it's not particularly necessary. If you've got a good quality primer simply apply it to the eye area as well when you're applying to the face. The upper lid is the most important part to primer as this is where much of your color is going to go. It will help the look last longer and help it go on smoother. Eyeliner is important for creating a dramatic look and it helps your eyes to pop but if you're blending correctly it should barely be noticeable.

Possibly one of the most overlooked secrets of eye makeup is to apply a highlight tone and luminizer to the inner eye. You can also add a light reflecting concealer to lift the area. The bright tone buried in the darkest part of the eye socket helps to make it pop.

You'll also want to curl your lashes before going any further. Heat the curler with a blow dryer but test it to make sure you don't get burned before applying. You want to curl your lashes before adding any mascara or other eye products because they could potentially cause your eye lashes to stick to the curler which would either mean having to straighten them carefully with a brush or that they could get pulled out.

Fake Lashes

99% of the time if you're admiring the sweep of a model's lashes it's because they are fake. Very few people have perfect, thick sweeping lashes.

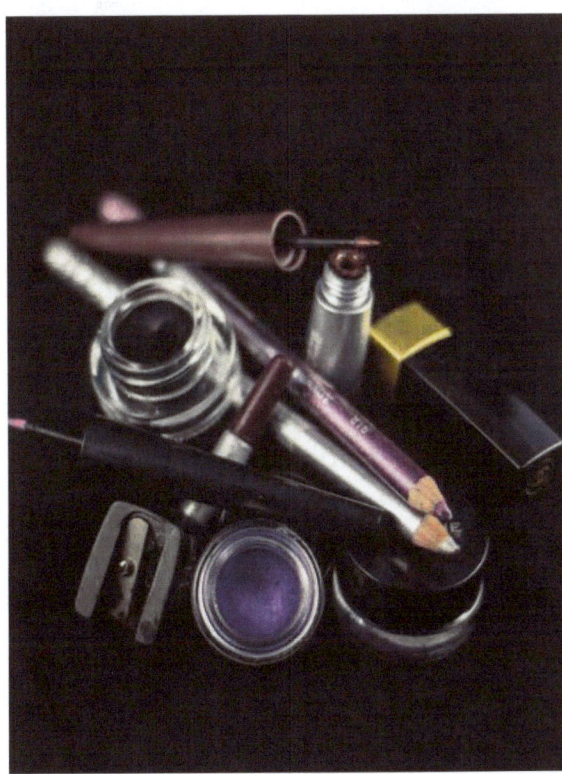

Mascara can only help so far. Individual false lashes are a much better choice than the full sets. They will give a far more natural look but if you're determined to have the full-length ones then you'll need to know about the different types. False lashes come in a variety of shapes, lengths, sizes and even have fun things like diamonds and feathers on the end if you're feeling courageous. If you're looking for doe eyes then choose ones that are longer in the middle, a sexy cat eyelash will be longer at one end. You'll want to find lashes that are only just somewhat longer than your own lashes if you're going for a look that is natural.

Place the lash above your lash line and trim so that it is a few millimeters inside the eye line from both ends. Before attaching curl the lashes so that they match your own. Make sure you do this before they're attached otherwise they are likely to spring loose. Apply the glue to the lashes – this is best done with a thin brush so that you don't end up with excess glue. Wait for 10-15 seconds before applying the lash to your skin so the glue can get tacky. Many people skip this step but it's imperative to getting a good, strong connection. Once they are applied you'll want to apply mascara to the whole thing to blend your lashes together with the false ones.

Catchy Eye Looks

Now that you've got the basics of color, shape, and brows down you can have some fun with them. Making a catchy eye look involves choosing proper colors for the look you want. However, there are some looks that have remained popular throughout. Here are a few looks with directions that you can have in your arsenal next time you need them. Apply your shadow and contouring before any false lashes, eyeliner, or mascara. A great tip for applying your mascara is to use the base of the handle from another brush (large powder brush works great) to stretch and lift the eyelid up so that you can get the mascara brush in there much easier.

White Contour

When it comes to contouring white is usually far too harsh a color. In fact, if you look at this color palette you're probably going to think it's far too harsh to ever work for anyone but a blue eyed or dark skinned person. In fact, it's a technique used by some of the top makeup artists so create a dramatic yet soft look.

Apply illuminating powder and then Bright White eyeshadow over the entire lid area, choose a shimmering white for an extra pop. Use dark gray to accent the crease and then apply a beige tone to the eyelid only. Above the gray fade a peach/pink tone into the brow area following the crease. Finish with a sweeping liner and a smudged line underneath.

Perfect Smoky Eye

There's no way around it, but this is one of the most fashionable eye makeup techniques around. There are so many ways to do the smoky eye that it's hard to pick just one that is the best. There's a fine line between smoky eyes and looking like a panda, which is why this is so hard despite being such a gorgeous look. The key to a perfect smoky eye is an understatement. You'll want to keep it as simple as possible to be successful.

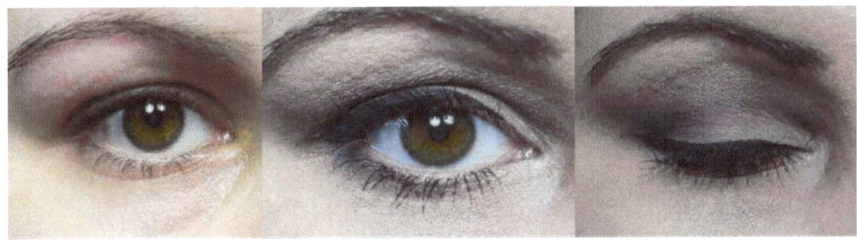

Tape a piece of scotch invisible tape (do not use medical tape or anything stronger as it will irritate the skin) against the upper lash line and out past the outer corner of your eye. Do not stick it down too hard, just gentle enough that it stays. You'll want to create a template line that you can follow extending to your brow from your nostril. Using a matte shadow and a large brush apply over the entire area a color similar to your iris or whatever tone you're trying to match (clothes etc). Add a dark gray shadow along the tape and above the crease of your eyelid. Do not put it past the center of your eye or make it too dark. Blend the gray in using a tone lighter than your skin color. Apply a black shadow on top of the outer edge of the gray shadow and gently blend in. Blend again using the lighter color. Line both top and bottom rims with a dark pencil. Start from the middle of the eye as this will make your eye appear larger. Remove the tape and apply a light, neutral shadow over the outside of the entire area to blend in.

The Winged Eyeliner

The key to doing a bold eyeliner is to understate your shadow. If you want your eyeliner to be the most noticeable feature of 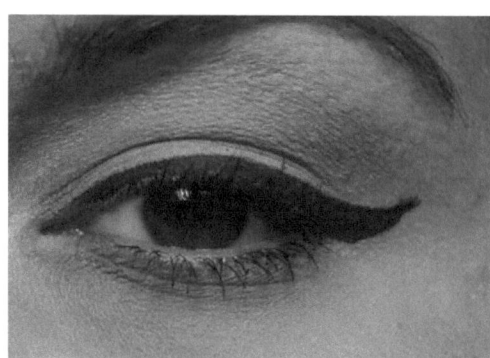 your eye makeup then you need it to stand out more than anything else. Winged eyeliner is the ultimate in simple yet classy looks yet if you're not painstaking with the line you'll look like you've got giant, black, chunky, blobs outside your eye. You'll want a liner pen or good control over your liner brush to achieve the sharp look needed, this isn't suitable for a pencil liner.

Start by creating a series of dots along the upper lid, starting from the tear duct. You'll want 5 dots along your lid then one below the end of the brow and then one between those two. Draw a line connecting the dots that curves at your tear duct and straightens towards the last 3 dots. Hold the handle of a spoon along the cheek up in a straight line from your eyebrow to the outer edge of your eye. From the outer edge of your eye draw a straight line up to where the dot is on the spoon and join them. Fill in the shape you have created solidly. Once your outline is filled in use a liquid liner and go over the entire shape to get a crisp line.

Chapter 6 – The Lips

You've probably decided you're just slapping some lipstick on and that's all at this point, but getting the perfect lip look takes work, and yes you can have perfect lips even if you're not Angelina Jolie-Pitt. The key to getting perfect lip shape is simply to fake it. In the same way that you've contoured your face and eyes, you can apply the technique to your lip area. The perfect lip shape is one that is balanced with the upper and lower lips being about the same size. As we age our lips thin so contouring can also make your face look more youthful with fuller lips. To avoid looking like a clown try not to overdo this, your lips aren't naturally huge but a little shape fixing doesn't hurt.

Lip Contouring

By now you should be familiar with highlights and shadows. The problem with just plain lipstick is that there are no highlights or shadows other than your own natural shape. It's a recipe for bland lips that don't have a wow factor. What you want is to add highlights and shadows to create a poutier appearance. This technique works regardless of color, you'll need to make sure your lips are hydrated and moisturized but if you've got an oily balm on top dab it off first. Lip primer is a good start, it will help the look last longer. Some people also exfoliate their lip skin but generally it's such a delicate area you shouldn't find this necessary.

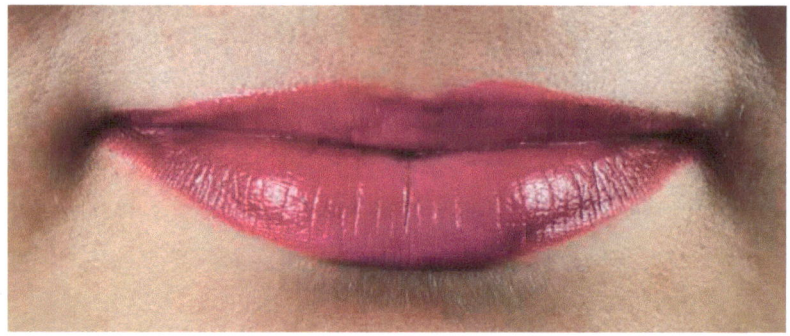

With a light toned nude pencil shade in the center of your lips as wide as your cupids bow. Remember you only want two shades lighter than the skin tone at most or you'll create an artificial look. The area should be about as wide as your finger. Using a darker lip pencil (use your darker skin color if you're going natural or two shades darker than your lipstick) outline the outer corners of your mouth with a soft line – about a finger width in. You don't want a hard line because it will make it more difficult to blend. Fill in the space like you did with the center. Blend the edges of both areas together using your fingertips. Using a lip brush apply your color in the area between where you just blended. Blend into both areas to create a lighter and darker shade. Using a dark pencil underline the middle of your bottom lip and blend upwards into the color. You can also do this with a brown eyeliner if this matches your skin tone, it will help create an extra shadow under your lips and make them seem bigger.

Adding a glossy topcoat can also help make lips look larger, especially if it's the lip plumping kind. Shiny lips tend to look fuller than matte. Similarly, you'll also want to avoid darker colors as these can thin your lips.

Make it Matte

Matte lipstick is very popular these days, but a lot of the good colors are expensive. You've probably got tons of lip colors that would work as matte tones or that you don't use because you don't like how glossy they are. There is a very simple technique to make any type or color of lipstick matte. You'll need your lips to be properly hydrated first, lipstick can dry the skin and make it flake off so this is essential to making your look last. Let the hydrator sit on your lip for several minutes before doing anything else. You'll have to touch-up using the same method if you want to reapply.

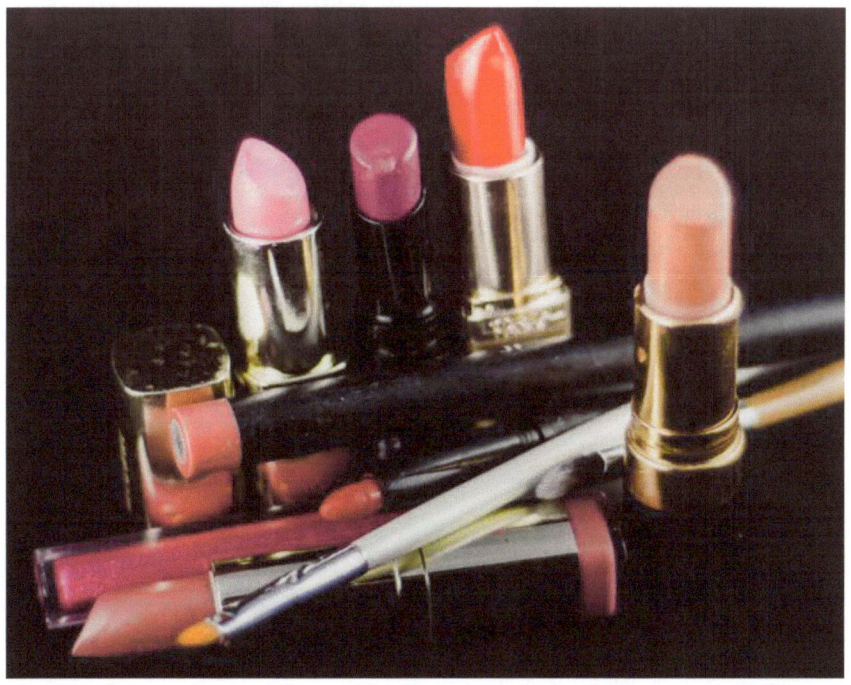

Using a lip liner that is similar in shade to the color you're using outline the whole lip and shade in towards the center. You can also use the contouring technique to make an ombre version too. Ombre is really popular and it looks impressive, but all that's been done is the same contouring as above and poof your lips have the perfect ombre. If you're going to ombre make sure you put primer on because you'll need the base layer to act as a blank canvas.

Outline the outside of your lips with a nude pencil to stop color bleeding and give a crisp edge. Apply your lipstick over the whole lip and over the top of the lip liner. Blot your lips so that they don't feel wet but the color is still there. Try and get it to look even. Using a translucent powder and a sponge pat the powder onto your lip gently. You'll want to apply a lot of powder to soak up the oils in the lipstick. Purse your lips and massage the powder in. Continue to apply powder if it doesn't seem matte enough yet. The only issue with this look is that the powder does not create a lot of staying power and it will come off fairly easily.

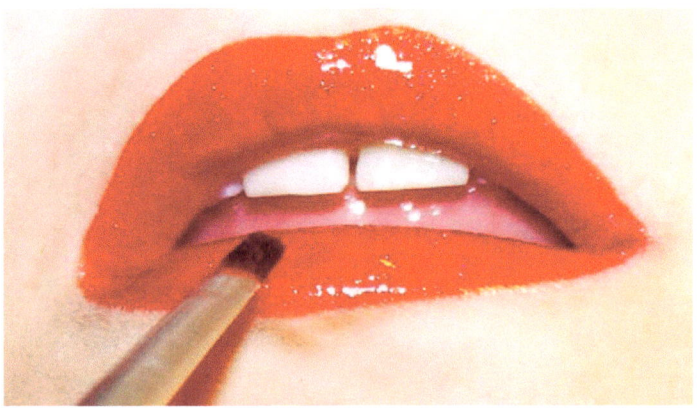

Making Lipstick Last

Many products these days are "guaranteed" to last through eating, all day, and never come off. Yet the majority of them still fall short of being perfection for long periods. If you're one of those people who struggles to keep their lipstick perfect through the day then you need these techniques. Using primer and a lip brush is much better for lasting color because it gets into the crannies of your lip much better than just swiping the tube over the top and helps to create a solid foundation for the color to stick to. Take your time and apply in layers rather than all at once. Most of the time lipstick comes off in layers, you'll still see your liner and a stain behind once your lipstick has mostly gone. To counteract this, you can simply blot your lips once you've finished your look (but before glossing) and then reapply another layer the same way. This will help add a second coat of color to make it last.

Conclusion

Thank you again for downloading this book!

I hope this book was able to help you to learn some new tricks to apply your makeup with perfection. Don't forget to take care of your skin from the inside first as this will help give you the perfect canvas to start your look.

Finally, if you enjoyed this book, please take the time to share your thoughts and post a review on Amazon. It'd be greatly appreciated!

Thank you and good luck!

www.ingramcontent.com/pod-product-compliance
Lightning Source LLC
Chambersburg PA
CBHW050829290526
45792CB00001B/319